How To Look Younger And Live Longer

317 Great Anti Aging And Life Extension Tips

ADAM COLTON

Published by BizMove
www.bizmove.com

Disclaimer

All the content found in this book was created for informational purposes only. The Content is not intended to be a substitute for professional medical advice, diagnosis, or treatment. Always seek the advice of your physician or other qualified health provider with any questions you may have regarding a medical condition. Never disregard professional medical advice or delay in seeking it because of something you have read in this book.

317 Great Anti Aging And Life Extension Tips

You want to find the best ways to ensure that you fight the effects of aging and remain feeling as young and vibrant as possible. It is important for your frame of mind for you to enjoy all that life has to offer. Follow the advice in this book if you want to keep that sense of youth.

1. Work with some weights to keep yourself looking younger. A toned body is a young body no matter what the chronological age may say. Working with the appropriate weights for your health will help you keep your body toned and looking fit, which will take years off of your body and soul.

2. When thinking about your aging process, if you are moved to be emotional, be emotional and then let it go. Don't mull over it. Aging can be tough, and tears will happen. Make a big effort to just move on to the next thing in your amazing life. This will help keep you positive and motivated.

3. If you want a tasty way to reduce the risk of osteoporosis, try adding soy to your diet. Soy contains calcium and plant estrogens which help prevent the loss of bone density. You can use

soy flour in your favorite recipes, snack on soy nuts, or use soy milk and cheeses.

4. Feel free to have a drink and a good meal once in a while. Even if you are watching your diet closely and do not consume alcohol on a regular basis, you should take the time to have a good glass of wine that you used to love and a great meal that was your favorite. Enjoy things in life.

5. As you get age, so does your brain. Studies have shown that exercising your brain is as important as exercising your body. Memory exercises will improve the mind and help stave off memory illness or dementia. Small exercises like memorizing 10 objects as you take a walk through your neighborhood, then writing them down when you get home is a good example to the mind nimble and alert.

6. A great way to minimize the effects of aging is to exercise your body but also your mind. There are fun and easy ways to exercise your brain daily, some of these ways include: crossword puzzles, word search puzzles, reading, crafts or any kind of hobby that will challenge your mind. By exercising your mind you are helping your body maintain its memory, which as well know is important as we age.

7. Try having a glass of red wine with dinner each night. There's a chemical found in red wine called resveratrol that has excellent anti-aging properties. But remember you should only drink alcohol in moderation. Drinking a moderate amount of red wine has also been shown to reduce your risk for heart problems.

8. Change your oils and change your life! Aging should mean less of the bad oils like partially hydrogenated, corn, cottonseed or soybean and more of the good like fish oil, flax oil, olive oil and nut oils! It is a painless change over that can really make a big difference in your overall health and well being, especially as you get older.

9. Take aspirin every day to prevent cardiac arrest, or "heart attacks". Heart attacks become more of a risk as you get older, and taking one aspirin a day has been found to help avoid them. Check with your doctor first to make sure that an aspirin regimen is safe for you.

10. At the end of the night, do not forget to wash off the makeup on your skin and around your eyes. This is very important, as you always want to give your skin the chance to breathe so that you can look fresh in the morning. Develop a

routine and designate a time at night to wash off your makeup.

11. Getting plenty of calcium will help you live longer and keep your bones healthy. When there is not enough calcium in your body, it will take the calcium from your bones. Over the years the bones will become weak and brittle which leads to fractures and osteoporosis. If you do not have enough calcium in your diet, consider taking a calcium supplement.

12. Make sure that you are getting enough calcium in your diet by eating more calcium-rich foods or by taking a supplement. As you age, your bones can lose calcium and become brittle. Brittle bones mean you can get a serious fracture from just a moderate bump. Fractures also do not heal as quickly as you age.

13. Cholesterol is a killer, so take the steps to lower your cholesterol. We absorb cholesterol not only from the foods we eat, but genes can pass high cholesterol also. For a longer life, go to your doctor and have your cholesterol checked and take any medications prescribed. Diet, exercise, and medications can all contribute to getting your cholesterol in check.

14. In order to decrease the wrinkles around your eyes, try using an anti-aging cream. The ingredients found in these creams have been proven to help eliminate and keep wrinkles away. You can put a small amount of cream on your fingers and rub it in a circular motion, gently around your wrinkles.

15. The aging process causes sleep quality to diminish. Even though you might not realize it, many diseases, such as heart disease and depression, can be attributed to poor sleep. To maintain optimum health, it is recommended that you get at least, seven to nine hours of sleep, each and every night. Making sure you get enough sleep is a positive step that you can take to help you look and feel great, at any age.

16. Aging is a worry for many people, but can be slowed down by remaining healthy. Daily exercise and a healthy diet can reduce aging effects, especially by drinking water. Getting plenty of sleep and taking care of your skin is another way to make sure you reduce wrinkles. Everyone ages, but that doesn't mean you can't age well!

17. Make sure you are eating REAL whole grains to help your body get the nutrients that it needs.

Most whole grains that you see in the store have been processed to the point that they are not much better than a piece of white bread. Eating whole grains like oats, quinoa and brown rice will give you the vitamins, minerals and fiber you need to keep feeling your best.

18. Take the time each day to enjoy the simple things in life. It could be a simple flower growing in the garden, or a smile on a child's face. These things will give you joy and the more joy you have in your life, the more youthful you will feel throughout it.

19. Surround yourself with wonderful people. If you find that the people that you spend a majority of your time with are grouchy more often than they are happy, consider looking for a new group of friends to hang out with. Happiness is contagious and if you are surrounded by it, you are likely to be joyful as well.

20. In order to age gracefully, be sure to see your doctor regularly! Putting off appointments with your doctor could really be detrimental in your overall health. Regular checkups make is possible for your doctor to catch problems while they are small enough to fix. Save yourself a good bit of

time, money and grief by keeping those appointments.

21. Gradually increase the time and effort you dedicate to your exercise regimen. As you age, your body requires more physical activity to maintain its strength and flexibility. Try to do a half hour walk, five days a week. Try adding in strength exercises about two times a week. Having a routine like this will keep your body healthy, and make you less susceptible to problems associated with age.

22. Understand hormone imbalances and be sure to treat them. As you age, many of the more difficult challenges are caused by imbalances in your hormones. This includes issues like depression, insomnia and weight increases. Go to your doctor if you are feeling off in any way and have yourself tested. Doctors can put you on a plan for supplementing your hormones.

23. If you find that you are feeling lonely when you are at home, consider getting a pet. They are wonderful companions and will provide you with company when no one else is around. Be sure that you pick the pet that will work out the best for you. If you do not want to commit to just

one pet, consider being a foster home for animals in shelters.

24. Wonderful memories will be produced by getting out of the house and traveling. You may not have the budget or the health to go on long vacations but just getting out of the house and going to the mall, park or theater is going to make you feel like life is worth living.

25. Just because you aren't as young as you used to be, you can still create goals and work to get them done. Life is an ever-changing journey and shouldn't become boring. Setting goals for yourself will keep you motivated and active to see they are accomplished. The pride you feel when you have attained these goals will be insurmountable.

26. Staying properly hydrated has never been more important to you than now! Aging is hard on the body and providing it with plenty of water will help flush toxins, bring nutrients to cells, hydrate skin and make it easier on every function of your body! Most experts recommend about eight glasses of water each day, so drink up for healthier aging!

27. Surround yourself with positive people. Grumpy, grouchy people are hard to be around and can affect both your mood and your health. Weed out the negativity by distancing yourself from those who cause you unnecessary stress or heartache. You've come much too far to let others pull you down with their nonsense.

28. Maintain a positive attitude. You're only as old as you feel, and if you stay positive aging can be a wonderful time of your life. Make sure you start every day giving thanks for what you have in your life, and watch how much better the day is when you approach it happily.

29. As we age, we like to reminisce. While being reminiscent, do not let your mind take guilt trips. Instead, take a trip to a favorite vacation spot or the mall. Have a trip on a cruise ship to exotic ports. Travel to a foreign country you have always wanted to visit. Guilt trips take you nowhere. Remember, you cannot undo what has already been done, so guilt trips are useless.

30. Antioxidants are absolutely one of your best weapons against aging! It is a proven fact that antioxidants counteract the free radicals that are constantly working against your body and the good things you are trying to do with it. Get

plenty of antioxidants as you age, with dark vegetables and fruits like carrots, squash and spinach or blue and purple berries!

31. Sugar has been proven to have an aging affect. You don't have to cut it out of your life completely, but definitely cut back on it. It has been shown to actually reduce the lifespan in multiple studies. Stick with foods that are naturally sweet like fruits to help your sweet cravings.

32. When aging, there is nothing more important than your personal health. If you feel good, consider what you have been doing and find ways to continue the momentum. If you feel mediocre, look for ways you can personally improve your health. If you feel sick, seek help and do so right away.

33. Don't get swallowed up by guilt. Guilt is a big enemy to healthy aging. As humans live longer lives, there is more and more to look back on and regret. But the exact opposite is true, too. There are more and more things for you to reminisce about in a positive way, as well. Don't mull negatively over the past, as it can only hurt your health for the future.

34. It is natural to lose some abilities as we age. There is a point in time when someone cannot care for their self. When it gets to this point, you should consider looking into a nursing home. It may not be something we want to do, yet it is much safer than living alone unable to care for ourselves. Licensed and trained professionals can provide you with the health care that you need in these environments.

35. Just because you aren't as young as you used to be, you can still create goals and work to get them done. Life is an ever-changing journey and shouldn't become boring. Setting goals for yourself will keep you motivated and active to see they are accomplished. The pride you feel when you have attained these goals will be insurmountable.

36. Stay active during the aging process. Staying active helps your body, mind, and soul. It will help you to age gracefully. Many studies also show that remaining active can have a positive effect on your mental capacity, and may help to keep diseases like Alzheimer's at bay. Try to include activity as part of your daily routine.

37. Surround yourself with positive people. Grumpy, grouchy people are hard to be around

and can affect both your mood and your health. Weed out the negativity by distancing yourself from those who cause you unnecessary stress or heartache. You've come much too far to let others pull you down with their nonsense.

38. Using olive oil is a key to keep your body looking and feeling young. Olive oil is a versatile, delicious and healthy way to reap the benefits of good oil for your body. Over the years, oils have gotten a bad rap from nutritionists, but oils are essential for keeping a body healthy.

39. Be independent. It might be easier to start to let others do things for you, but to stay vibrant, maintain your sense of independence and your ability to do things for yourself as you get older. Not only will it keep you busy, but you stay strong as you do things for yourself.

40. Include more fiber in your diet by including more whole grains and vegetables as you become older. Your digestive system becomes more sensitive as you age, so it is important to make sure that the foods you eat are easily digested. Keeping your digestive system in good working order will prevent many health problems.

41. As your eyes age, you need to take care of them. At the age of 40, have a complete eye exam that will screen for glaucoma, fully measure the vision in each eye, and have your retinas tested for retinal damage. If the findings indicate, be sure to have an annual checkup to make sure that glaucoma or macular eye disease has not begun to show symptoms.

42. The next time you go to the store, look in the facial care section for anti-aging products. There are many creams and gels on the market that you can apply to your face that contain vitamin E, which can help to smooth and tone the surface of your skin. Improve your facial care and slow down the aging process with anti-aging products.

43. Have a screening done for Alzheimer's disease, especially if you are experiencing memory loss. Ability to remember things declines slightly with age, but if you have a family history of dementia and are having memory loss, get tested. There are medications available to slow the disease down, but you have to be diagnosed first.

44. A great way to slow the aging process and keep feeling young is to make health your hobby. Try keeping a journal of the foods you eat and evaluate it at the end of the week to see how

healthy you are eating and work on not only eating better but eating properly for a longer life.

45. A great tip to follow in order to achieve healthy aging is to stay positive. Studies show that people that are more positive towards life tend to live longer as compared to people who worry all the time. Try to add humor into your life and always remember to laugh.

46. Research suggests that one way to live a longer and healthier life is to form deep social connections. Do not under-estimate the therapeutic value of giving and receiving love. Make sure you make time in your daily schedule to enjoy and strengthen the love relationships in your life. If you have troubled relationships with family members, take the time and effort to heal them. By healing others, you start healing yourself and alleviate stress from your life.

47. Make sure you are eating REAL whole grains to help your body get the nutrients that it needs. Most whole grains that you see in the store have been processed to the point that they are not much better than a piece of white bread. Eating whole grains like oats, quinoa and brown rice will give you the vitamins, minerals and fiber you need to keep feeling your best.

48. Even if you have never had a massage in your life, go and get one on a regular basis. It is not only great for your body to get the blood flowing and the tense muscles relaxed, but it will also be good for the soul. It will feel great and leave you feeling wonderful and happy.

49. Faze out the junk food. You are what you eat, and eating junk will lead to a very unhealthy aging process. In fact, not shockingly, many studies show that humans that eat more pure, healthy foods live longer and healthier lives. Cut out the junk food and concentrate on choosing healthy alternatives.

50. Prepare for the end. If you take the time to prepare a living will and pre-plan your funeral you will find much peace in the process. Dying is a part of living that cannot be beat and having a plan that is ready for that time is a gift to yourself as well as the rest of your family.

51. Stay active during the aging process. Staying active helps your body, mind, and soul. It will help you to age gracefully. Many studies also show that remaining active can have a positive effect on your mental capacity, and may help to

keep diseases like Alzheimer's at bay. Try to include activity as part of your daily routine.

52. Do protect your skin against wrinkles and cancer by wearing proper sunblock but don't over do it to the extent that you deprive yourself of much needed vitamin D! As much harm as too much sun can do, too little of it can also hurt you so find a suitable SPF that will prevent damage without completely prohibiting your intake of highly beneficial sunlight!

53. A critical factor to prevent aging and increase lifespan is to not smoke. Smoking destroys the body and speeds up the aging process. Smoking is the easiest way to look older and shorten your lifespan at the same time. It causes disease, ages the skin, and is overall one of the main preventable killers known to man.

54. Sit down and have a nice cup of tea to slow the aging process. Drinking tea has two-fold benefits. First, tea has been shown to be chock full of antioxidants and cancer fighting compounds that help keep you healthy. Second, sitting down and having a cup of tea is a great stress reliever and good for your body and soul.

55. Sign up to a new class. It is never too late to learn something new, so consider attending some public lectures or joining a community class. Choose a topic you are interested it, whether it is computers, gardening, crafts, philosophy, foreign languages, or quantum physics. Continuous learning will stop your mind from being idle.

56. Find a support group if you're having trouble adjusting to age. Other people who are going through the same things you're going through may have different ways of doing things and different methods of coping. They can help you navigate the unfamiliar waters of aging as well as lend an ear or shoulder to lean on.

57. Focus on your support network as you age to prevent a sense of loneliness or isolation. Spend time with your friends and family whenever possible, whether it is a lunch date or a chat on the telephone. Connecting with your family and friends can serve to offset depression or loneliness, especially as your personal family situation may be changing.

58. If you want to reduce the effects of aging, be sure that you get plenty of rest. Not only is it good for your overall body, it also helps to give

you the energy boost that you need. Taking a one hour nap is also a good idea, too.

59. Aging causes changes in your digestive system. Constipation is a more common problem in older adults that younger ones. A combination of factors can contribute to constipation, including low fluid intake, a low-fiber diet, and not enough exercise. To help prevent constipation, drink plenty of fluids, include plenty of fruits, vegetables and whole grains in your diet. You should also include more physical activities in your daily routine.

60. Birds of a feather flock together, so carefully consider the people you spend the most time with. Are they helping or hurting you? People who are grumpy will drag you down, so spend more time with the upbeat friends you have to keep yourself in good spirits.

61. Stress is a big factor in aging, so be sure to keep your body balanced and calm. Exercising about 20 minutes daily is a great way to retain inner peace and to be healthier.

62. As you get older you may find that you enjoy the simple things in life more and more. Appreciate the beauty of nature, the flavors of food, or the

joy of a good hug. This will keep your heart warm and your mind free of worry, which can help slow the aging process.

63. Whiten your teeth to take some serious years off of your age. Years of drinking coffee and wine and smoking can do a serious number of the appearance of our teeth. Shave off some years by having your teeth professionally whitened. The difference it makes will astound you.

64. Go for regular preventive health check-ups with your local physician. As you get older, your body is more susceptible to disease and injury. By having regular check-ups, you could detect and treat small health problems before they turn into bigger problems. It is also recommended that you attend dental and eyes check-ups as well.

65. One of the first things to start going when you age is your eyesight. As you age, it begins to rapidly deteriorate. Make sure that as you age you have frequent visits to the ophthalmologist, in order to track your eyes' degradation, and have glasses or contacts prescribed in order to make it less drastic.

66. To make sure you are getting a proper amount of nutrients in your life as you age, try drinking

smoothies, three to four times each week. Smoothies taste great and are chock full of good things. They typically contain up to five nutritional servings of fruits and vegetables. Even better, smoothies are rather filling, so as a light lunch or a snack, they can help you control your cravings and lose weight!

67. You should enjoy your journey through your life. If you make time to enjoy the milestones in life as you did with your children as they got older, you will be able to feel the same way they did when you reach them.

68. Simplify the things in your life. Start with your bedroom closet, and go from there. Eliminate the many things that you do not use. You will quickly see that many of the things around your house are just clutter and serve absolutely no purpose in your life. De-cluttering will lessen the stress in your life.

69. As you get older, keeping a good balance when walking is a common complaint. Oftentimes, some may resort to using a walker or cane to help them keep their footing. Studies had shown that instead of using the customary walker or cane, instead, use a pole. A pole will help

strengthen the upper body as well as help the balance of the senior when they walk.

70. A critical factor to prevent aging and increase lifespan is to not smoke. Smoking destroys the body and speeds up the aging process. Smoking is the easiest way to look older and shorten your lifespan at the same time. It causes disease, ages the skin, and is overall one of the main preventable killers known to man.

71. Try moving around more and sitting still less. Especially if you're retired and aren't moving around for work any more. Try taking up a hobby that involves moving around - golf is a particularly good once since it's not a high impact sport but it keeps you moving. Studies have shown that getting up and moving can help you keep your blood pressure levels in normal ranges and lower your risk for heart problems.

72. If you notice a lack of balance, weakened limbs, memory loss and poor coordination as you age, start taking a vitamin B12 supplement. Most people automatically assume that senility is the cause of memory loss yet it can also be a vitamin B12 deficiency. Talk to your doctor about testing to see if you are vitamin B12 deficient and how much you should supplement into your diet.

73. In order to keep the signs of aging at bay, you need to avoid overeating and stuffing yourself until full. Do not starve yourself, but there is no better way to slow aging and extend life than cutting back on the calories. Just as a rule of thumb, avoid overeating in any situation.

74. Keep up with your social calendar as you age. Studies have shown that people with an active social life have less chance of suffering from Alzheimer's. Visiting with friends and family will nourish those relationships and keep your mental health in top condition. Sharing your life with your social circle will lead you to a more fulfilling life.

75. Many people gain weight as they age. Keeping an ideal weight cuts the risk of a number of health problems ranging from diabetes, stroke, and a plethora of cancers. You will be able to lose fat and stay thin, thanks to a better diet and exercise.

76. Eating organic foods can significantly reduce irritation issues due to food consumption. These foods have fewer chemicals and such on them, which allows you to be eating more all natural foods. This will take away much skin irritation

from eating those other foods, and it will help you in your aging process.

77. Keeping your skin healthy aids the aging process. It is never too soon to begin protecting your skin by avoiding damaging UV rays. Being out in the sun too long without protection can advance the formation of wrinkles as well as skin cancer.

78. Enjoy the time you get after retirement! Engage in activities you enjoy with the people you love and you'll find your heart is stronger and your mind is clearer. Being happy goes along with being healthy and the more you do to keep your spirits high, the slower the aging process will become.

79. Taking care of your skin at an early age will play a large role in how you look as you age. Remember to always use sunscreen when you are out in the sun, and dress appropriately for the weather. Use moisturizers and lotions to protect your skin and keep yourself looking healthy.

80. To help your mindset while aging, toss out any numbers that aren't really important, specifically your weight, your height and most importantly your age. These numbers may be important for

your doctor (and they should be), but for daily living they are just barriers to the many, many things that are possible for you to do.

81. Living can be very hard work. Even if you do not have a job outside of the home, it is going to take it out of you some days. Take the time to rest now and then. You could do this every day if your schedule permits but if it does not, be sure to rest and relax at least a couple times a week.

82. Faze out the junk food. You are what you eat, and eating junk will lead to a very unhealthy aging process. In fact, not shockingly, many studies show that humans that eat more pure, healthy foods live longer and healthier lives. Cut out the junk food and concentrate on choosing healthy alternatives.

83. To help slow the process of aging, try to stay as active as possible, for your given circumstance. Sitting idly, will speed up muscular decay and before you know it, you will be stuck with a sedentary lifestyle. Even a lap around the block would be beneficial.

84. Oral health is essential to a long life. Even if you do not have teeth anymore, it is still important to go and have regular exams at the dentist so he

can check your gums. You can still develop gum disease, oral cancer and other things that can lead to other health problems.

85. Get the proper amount of water each day! This is important as the years go by! Without proper hydration, your body will react in terrible ways. It could lead to things as serious as seizures, brain damage or even death. Buy a large jug that will hold eight glasses of water and fill it each morning. Make sure that it is empty by the time you go to bed.

86. Most everyone is lacking one vitamin or another, but one vitamin that most people, especially those that are aging don't get enough of is Vitamin D. Vitamin D helps your internal health as well as your well-being, so to age gracefully, begin by getting a little sunlight each day, which is the best source of Vitamin D. It is also acceptable to supplement with foods high in Vitamin D as well as vitamin supplements.

87. Learn something new. There's an old saying that says, "you can't teach an old dog new tricks"; it's a myth. Get out there and take a class or develop a hobby. Not only will it occupy your time. Your brain will get a workout from the new information you're learning.

88. A tip for staying young, even when your body is aging, is to keep learning. Learn more about playing bridge, how to use a computer, gardening, woodworking, or whatever you wanted to learn earlier in life but didn't have the time to do. Since you are retired and your children are grown, you no longer have the excuse of not having the time to delve into these new adventures of learning. Never let your brain remain idle!

89. Consider taking health supplements to make sure you're getting adequate nutrition and vitamins. Investigate different health supplements and talk to your doctor to determine whether your health would benefit from the use of some supplementation. There are many good supplements available to help you make sure that your health stays great.

90. Stay flexible. Muscle and skeletal problems are linked to lack of flexibility, so make sure to do some stretching at least three days a week. Breathe normal throughout each stretch and hold it for 10-30 seconds. Stretching will help your body stay loose and supple so that it doesn't feel tight and stiff.

91. Revisiting an old hobby is an excellent way to help you occupy time as a retiree or empty nester. It will help you to enjoy positive things as your lifestyle changes with age. After all, when you no longer have to work or do not have as much time wrapped up in raising a family, you can focus on interests you may have neglected over the years. Hobbies not only keep you active but also fill those times when you may feel lonely or overwhelmed with what to do with yourself.

92. Make sure you prepare for an emergency. As you age you can't move as quickly as you did when you were younger, and it might take you longer to get things together or remember things in a pinch. Have some things in place for when there's an emergency and you need to act fast.

93. An aspirin a day will keep the doctor at bay, and also help you reduce the risk of heart attack for a longer life. The American Heart Association now recommends a low-dose of aspirin for patients who have had a previous heart attack, are in high risk classes for heart attack, and those who have unstable angina. Consult your doctor to find out if aspirin is right for you to lead a longer life.

94. As one ages, it is important to supply the body with the nutrients it needs to regain or maintain

optimum health. One way to make sure that your body has all the nutrients it needs is to take proper nutritional supplements. Some supplements you may wish to consider are multi-vitamins, anti-inflammatories, and anti-oxidants. Remember to seek the advice of your physician before taking any new supplements.

95. As we age, everyday things such as bending over to pick things up or everyday activities like putting groceries in the car can become painful chores. Pain from arthritis and many other effects of aging can really make life difficult. While you are working on diet, supplementation and fitness to alleviate the condition, don't be afraid to ask for help while shopping or doing other everyday chores. You deserve it!

96. When aging, there is nothing more important than your personal health. If you feel good, consider what you have been doing and find ways to continue the momentum. If you feel mediocre, look for ways you can personally improve your health. If you feel sick, seek help and do so right away.

97. Step up your workout routine. As you get older, your body requires more time and energy to maintain its strength and flexibility. Try walking

quickly for 30 minutes, five days per week. Round out the week with two days of doing strength exercises. This will help you stay in great shape and avoid early aging issues so many people deal with.

98. One of the hardest things to manage for the person who is aging and for those around him or her is dementia. If someone you love, has dementia be as patient as possible with them. Often, they don't know the severity of their own condition. To help your own spirits, take their dementia as a mercy, as it must be hard to die having all your memories intact.

99. When you get older, you tend to want to hold onto the past and resist change, but you should really embrace this change as the whole part of the process of getting older. It's all in the attitude. Look forward to them, and think of them as a new adventure.

100. To make sure you are getting a proper amount of nutrients in your life as you age, try drinking smoothies, three to four times each week. Smoothies taste great and are chock full of good things. They typically contain up to five nutritional servings of fruits and vegetables. Even better, smoothies are rather filling, so as a

light lunch or a snack, they can help you control your cravings and lose weight!

101.   One solid piece of advice for to maintain good health as you are aging is to eat a balanced diet. A diet which is well-balanced includes meals rich in vegetables, fruits, and whole grains. Make sure you limit your intake of trans fat, saturated fats and cholesterol. By eating a well-balanced diet, your body is supplied the essential nutrients it needs to maintain optimum health.

102.   If you want to keep looking young, laugh! And do it often! Watch funny TV shows, read jokes on the internet, or go see a comedian. Make sure you include daily doses of laughter. Laughing will keep you looking young, and can also extend your life.

103.   Surround yourself with positive people. Grumpy, grouchy people are hard to be around and can affect both your mood and your health. Weed out the negativity by distancing yourself from those who cause you unnecessary stress or heartache. You've come much too far to let others pull you down with their nonsense.

104.   Aging gracefully is everyone's goal in life. A great way to start on that path is adopt a healthy

diet - and it's never too late to start. By eating five fruits and vegetables, at least three servings of whole grains, and drinking five to eight glasses of eight ounce water a day, you will be giving your body the proper nutrients it needs to begin the aging process gracefully. There are many easy ways to get fruits and vegetables too - have you tried juicing?

105.   Stay close to your family and friends. They are the people who will take care of you as you get older, but more than that: they are the ones that love you. Cultivate and nurture those relationships as you age so that you get even closer as time goes on.

106.   Be independent. It might be easier to start to let others do things for you, but to stay vibrant, maintain your sense of independence and your ability to do things for yourself as you get older. Not only will it keep you busy, but you stay strong as you do things for yourself.

107.   As you age, do not forget to block out the sun! Keep applying sunscreen. This will help your age spots stay small and not enlarge or keep multiplying. Wear sunscreen every day, even in the winter. This will help keep your skin youthful and diminish the appearance of age spots.

108.   Alzheimer's disease is a common disease. Recognizing it early is the best defense in slowing the disease down. The likelihood of getting Alzheimer's disease increases with risk factors as having a family history of the disease, Down's Syndrome, serious head injury in the past or being over 65 years of age.

109.   Have the seasonal flu vaccine every year. As you get older, you will become more susceptible to illnesses, including the flu. The flu can also do more damage on an older body. So to stay healthy throughout that November-April flu season, have a flu shot every year, preferably in September or October.

110.   Protect yourself from fraud. Con artists often target older people who can be vulnerable or too trusting. Protect your identity by withholding your personal banking information whenever possible, destroying documents with your personal data and limiting access to your home to include only known individuals. Being cautious will help you keep your money out of the hands of scammers.

111.   Work with some weights to keep yourself looking younger. A toned body is a young body

no matter what the chronological age may say. Working with the appropriate weights for your health will help you keep your body toned and looking fit, which will take years off of your body and soul.

112.   If you want to age gracefully, then you should try to do something you like every day. By doing this, you will get fulfillment out of each and every day because you are doing something that you look forward to, which keeps you motivated to continue and keeps the enjoyment flowing.

113.   Depression is a "hidden" risk for developing osteoporosis. Cortisol is a stress-related hormone related to depression that depletes the bones of minerals. Studies have shown that women with depression have lower bone density in their spines and hips. So, if you're feeling down, see your doctor to find out if you have depression.

114.   For healthy aging, consider grazing over six smaller meals, instead of three big ones. Studies have shown that this helps your body absorb more nutrients, control its weight and decrease the potential for heartburn. In fact, some studies have shown that eating the same amount of

calories in six smaller meals has led to considerable weight loss!

115.   As you age, to continue to have healthy looking skin moisturize it every day. How your skin looks is directly related to the amount of moisture your skin is receiving. It's important then to get moisture back into the skin, so choose a moisturizer that works best for you and use it daily. This is an area related to aging that you can have a significant impact on.

116.   Maintain your muscle mass by getting exercise on a regular basis. Use a pedometer and make sure that you are taking at least 5,000 to 10,000 steps each day. If you maintain your muscle mass, you are sure to avoid some of the terrible falls that you would otherwise incur.

117.   You must maintain a healthy body weight into your golden years. If you are overweight there are obvious health risks that you face but there are equally dangerous risks involved with being underweight. Talk with your doctor to learn what your ideal weight is and strive to reach that weight.

118.   Just because you are aging doesn't mean you should just sit back and take it easy. To maintain

good health, you need to continue to be as active as you possibly can. Sure, you may not be able to go out and race in a marathon, but you still can incorporate some activity into you daily activities. It is suggested that you include at least 30 minutes of physical activity each day. Maybe you could take a 15-minute walk twice a day. Dust off that old bike and take a ride around the neighborhood.

119.   One of the main contributing factors to a shorter life is the amount of sugar we eat. The aging process is accelerated and your lifespan reduced with excessive sugar consumption. This link between sugar and reduced lifespan has been studied and clearly proven.

120.   Want to live a long life and enjoy the aging process? To live longer, stay positive. Studies have demonstrated that those who have a positive attitude also tend to have a longer and healthier life. Look for the humor in life. Laughter can lower that high blood pressure and help drain the stress right out of your body. Numerous studies have shown the positive powers of laughter and how it makes you feel better.

121.   Surround yourself with positive people. Grumpy, grouchy people are hard to be around and can affect both your mood and your health. Weed out the negativity by distancing yourself from those who cause you unnecessary stress or heartache. You've come much too far to let others pull you down with their nonsense.

122.   Each night, sleep a minimum of 7 to 9 hours. Insufficient sleep can lead to diseases from depression to heart disease, and has been linked to cancer. Exercise helps. Some doctors recommend melatonin (a hormone produced in humans by the pineal gland) or L-theanine, an amino acid found in tea. See an age management physician for healthy sleeping advice.

123.   Adding green tea to your daily routine can really boost your anti-aging regimen! Green tea can help build your resistance against many diseases such as cancer and can also defend you against dementia and other neurological ailments of aging. Also of note, green tea can assist your body in its ability to burn fat, so making it a permanent addition to your grocery list is a very good idea!

124.   If you notice a lack of balance, weakened limbs, memory loss and poor coordination as

you age, start taking a vitamin B12 supplement. Most people automatically assume that senility is the cause of memory loss yet it can also be a vitamin B12 deficiency. Talk to your doctor about testing to see if you are vitamin B12 deficient and how much you should supplement into your diet.

125.   Eat well and healthily. Eating lots of fruits, vegetables, and whole wheats can help you against signs of aging and keep your body strong and protected. Also, drink a lot of water, up to eight glases a day. Finally, you should try to watch the amount of fat you eat. Keep the daily calories you get from fat under 35% and it should help you keep your body shape.

126.   Keep your body fit and functioning at its peak, even while growing older. Exercising is not just for weight loss, it is also incredibly important for keeping your body young and working at its optimum level. Cardio exercise is extremely important for your heart health, so keep your body moving to keep the years away.

127.   Use olive oil and remember fat does not equal bad. Oils have gotten a bad rap in the past few decades but oils are essential to our health. The trick is to stay away from "fake" fats like

trans fats. The use of olive oil has many heart healthy benefits so don't shy away from using it. Try making your own salad vinaigrette's of olive oil and balsamic vinegar.

128.   Exercise can improve the aging process. As we get older, our muscle mass naturally declines, making everyday activities more difficult and reducing the number of calories we burn. While aerobic exercise helps maintain muscle mass and control weight, resistance exercise has the added benefit of helping maintain bone mass.

129.   Join senior groups, church groups local government groups or hobby clubs. Build a family unit, even if your blood relatives are not near you. It's important to have a network of people around you as you age. Your friends and family can cheer you up during hard times and be your sounding board or first warning signal during bad times. If your family is far away, look to your community.

130.   You must get plenty of calcium to aid in the prevention of osteoporosis. Milk, skim milk, yogurt, and low-fat cheeses can be good ways to get calcium. Broccoli contains a large amount of calcium as well as other veggies. And take your

calcium supplements. Women need 1500 to 2000 mg after menopause and men after the age of 65.

131.   Take a computer course or have someone teach you the basics of the internet. It can take you places that you may never see in your life. It is like a vacation or a journey that you can take from the comfort of your own home. There are so many things that you will learn while on the internet.

132.   Do not let others make you feel as if you are less of a person now than you were in your youth. You may require more care from others than you used to but you are just as important and it is crucial that you remember who you were and who you are for the rest of your life.

133.   Keep up with the golden rule to treat others as you would like them to treat you. Even though many people think that many of the elderly are mean and grumpy, you do not have to be that way. Treat others with the respect and sensitivity that you would like them to treat you and you are sure to get the same in return.

134.   A key element to staying young and looking young is to get plenty of sleep. Not only is it important on how you look each day, but it is

critical to feeling your best. Everyone's ideal amount of sleep is different so determine when you feel best after different lengths of sleep over a week.

135.   Maintain a positive attitude. You're only as old as you feel, and if you stay positive aging can be a wonderful time of your life. Make sure you start every day giving thanks for what you have in your life, and watch how much better the day is when you approach it happily.

136.   Doing lots of cardiovascular exercise will keep you fit and help you feel younger. Cardiovascular exercise is important for vascular health and gets the blood pumping to make you feel good. A good schedule for cardiovascular exercise is to do 40 minutes every other day to increase heart health and make you feel good.

137.   As you become older you will start to find parts of your body not working as well as they used to. For some things, it is possible to take medication but for others, you will simply have to accept these facts. It can be hard to accept but the faster you do the easier it will be for you.

138.   Write your life story down. It doesn't have to be a major novel, but create some account of

your life so that your children or grandchildren can get to know all of the things you've seen and gone through during your life. No children? Do it for relatives or friends.

139.   If you notice a lack of balance, weakened limbs, memory loss and poor coordination as you age, start taking a vitamin B12 supplement. Most people automatically assume that senility is the cause of memory loss yet it can also be a vitamin B12 deficiency. Talk to your doctor about testing to see if you are vitamin B12 deficient and how much you should supplement into your diet.

140.   Instead of driving everywhere that you go, take a walk to the shop if you are within a mile. This will provide you with additional flexibility, which will be very important to your joints for combating the signs of aging. Keep the car in the garage for a day and take advantage of the weather in your area.

141.   Tell your doctor about the medications you take. Bring a list of all prescription and non-prescription drugs, supplements, herbs and vitamins including dosage. If it's easier, bring the bottles. Your doctor should say if they are okay or have potentially bad interactions. As you age,

you'll have an increasing chance of having bad side effects from medications, including those that are non-prescription or over-the-counter.

142.	Keeping your weight under control is one key to aging well. There are a number of ailments related to obesity which exacerbate age-related illnesses. In order to keep your weight under control, you should exercise moderately and eat a balanced diet. Tracking your food intake with an online food diary makes this easier.

143.	When thinking about your aging process, if you are moved to be emotional, be emotional and then let it go. Don't mull over it. Aging can be tough, and tears will happen. Make a big effort to just move on to the next thing in your amazing life. This will help keep you positive and motivated.

144.	It may sound depressing but remember you are nearing the end of your life each day. Keeping this in mind will allow you to appreciate even the smallest things in life. It will give you the drive to strive to get the most out of each and every day in your life.

145.	As you age, your skin needs more care since it is aging also. When outdoors, you need to protect your skin from the harmful rays emitted by the sun. You should apply a sunscreen with a sun protection factor (SPF) which is at least a 15. Spending too much time in the sun without proper sun protection can also lead to those unwanted, dark age spots which are associated with aging skin.

146.   Go out with friends and family. One of the worst things to do as you start to get older is to isolate yourself in your home. Make sure you get out a few times a week for anything: to volunteer, to have lunch or any of hundreds of possibilities. Going out and seeing others has a great effect on your mental health.

147.   A critical factor to prevent aging and increase lifespan is to not smoke. Smoking destroys the body and speeds up the aging process. Smoking is the easiest way to look older and shorten your lifespan at the same time. It causes disease, ages the skin, and is overall one of the main preventable killers known to man.

148.   A good way to reduce the impact of lines around the eyes is to wear sunglasses. Not only does this prevent squinting and causing crows feet, but sunglasses block the sun from hitting those high wrinkle areas and damaging the skin.

So wearing sunglasses has a dual effect on the anti-aging process.

149.   Sit down and have a nice cup of tea to slow the aging process. Drinking tea has two-fold benefits. First, tea has been shown to be chock full of antioxidants and cancer fighting compounds that help keep you healthy. Second, sitting down and having a cup of tea is a great stress reliever and good for your body and soul.

150.   Doing lots of cardiovascular exercise will keep you fit and help you feel younger. Cardiovascular exercise is important for vascular health and gets the blood pumping to make you feel good. A good schedule for cardiovascular exercise is to do 40 minutes every other day to increase heart health and make you feel good.

151.   To stave off memory problems, try incorporating exercise into your day. Exercise will decrease the chance of getting dementia in older adults by 60% percent. Exercise increases the flow of oxygen to the brain, which in turn strengthens the brain's neurons that are related to memory and learning. So, exercising the body is also exercising the mind.

152.   During the course of the day, act silly and joke around with friends and family. The more that you joke, the lower your heart rate will be and the better you will feel as the day wears on. This can go a long way in reducing your stress and helping you to become more beautiful.

153.   Make sure that when you are eating, you are putting essential fatty acids into your body. These are imperative for cell growth and maintaining the proper blood pressure so you are not at risk for any diseases. Also, essential fatty acids can go a long way in improving your cholesterol level and reducing aging symptoms.

154.   Learning how to physically intake your food in a beneficial way is a key element to eating right. Eat half as much as you normally do, and eat twice as often. Also chew your food for twice as long as you normally would. This will curb hunger, help improve nutrition absorption, and help control your weight.

155.   A good anti-aging tip is restoring your hormones. As you age, your declining hormone levels cause symptoms, such as loss of energy and stamina, a flagging libido and sleep issues. It would likely be helpful for you to talk with a doctor about hormone therapy.

156.   Stay positive about life and growing older. Just because you are getting older does not mean that your life has to end and stop right there. A good thing to do is to stay active with social activities and keep friends and family in your life. You will be happy you did.

157.   With aging, our bones tends to decrease in size and they lose density. This causes your bones to weaken which makes them more apt to fracture easily. Because of these two changes to the bone tissue, people tend to become shorter in stature as they age. To combat these changes in your bones, include plenty of vitamin D and calcium in your diet. You can build bone density by doing weight-bearing activities such as walking.

158.   If you wish to stay wrinkle free, avoid frowning. While humorous, it's true. If you find yourself frowning, give yourself a sharp pinch. In time, you will break the habit.

159.   Grab a fashionable pair of sunglasses and wear them. Wearing a cute pair of glasses can help with looking younger but the biggest benefit is the protection it gives to your eyes and skin. The skin around our eyes is very thin and the

suns UV rays can do a number on that area. Wearing glasses with that protect from uv rays will keep your skin protected and your eyes bright.

160.   To slow down the aging process, do some aerobic exercise everyday mixed with occasional light weight training. Numerous scientific studies have shown that exercise improves muscle strength, stamina, bone density and balance. As these four things deteriorate with age, regular exercise could help keep your body in good condition well into your 80s and beyond.

161.   While you are aging, be sure to maintain a balanced diet. Thinking about a balanced diet isn't just for your younger years. In fact, it is more important as you age. Make sure your body is getting the proper amount of fiber, vegetables, fruits, cholesterols and fats. Being proactive on this will help you keep up your health for a long time.

162.   A positive attitude is important as you age. If you can make someone else smile, you will smile yourself. It does not cost anything to spread happiness. It is also priceless when given to others.

163.   If you find that you are feeling lonely when you are at home, consider getting a pet. They are wonderful companions and will provide you with company when no one else is around. Be sure that you pick the pet that will work out the best for you. If you do not want to commit to just one pet, consider being a foster home for animals in shelters.

164.   Keep up with the latest styles. Although some of today's fashion is a bit off the wall, you are sure to find a piece or two that you will feel comfortable wearing. Just by adding a trendy top to your outfit, you are sure to feel and look good and the younger generations will notice.

165.   Even if your body is deteriorating, you do not have to let your spirit deteriorate as well. Keep growing as a person through reading books, sharing stories with loved ones or enjoying a good old movie now and then. Keep your youthful spirit alive as long as you live.

166.   Maintain your muscle mass by getting exercise on a regular basis. Use a pedometer and make sure that you are taking at least 5,000 to 10,000 steps each day. If you maintain your muscle mass, you are sure to avoid some of the terrible falls that you would otherwise incur.

167.   Eating fish is a great way to slow the aging process and stay young. A lot of new evidence is suggesting that beneficial elements, such as omega-3 fatty acids, are excellent for the skin. Even people who do not like fish can reap the benefits from it by taking a fish oil supplement.

168.   Start making a will. Death is a topic people don't like to talk about, but it is inevitable. When you feel ready, begin preparing your will and final papers so that your family knows how you would like things to be handled after you pass on. This will also make sure that there are not any family fights and disagreements later on.

169.   As you start getting older, your metabolism slows down. So if you aren't at a weight you are comfortable with now, it will be even harder to keep your weight under control as you age. Take up exercise and get moving regularly, preferably 3 to 4 days a week.

170.   You need to make sure your eyes have adequate protection as you age. The eye ages along with every other part of your body. Protect your eyes against ultraviolet radiation by wearing sunglasses with a high UV rating every time you

leave the house. Regular drugstore sunglasses are acceptable only if they contain a high UV rating.

171.   Make sure that you visit your doctor regularly for a check-up as you get older. Issues like high blood pressure, high cholesterol and mobility issues need to be monitored more frequently because your body will take longer to recover from health problems. Your doctor can advise you if you need to change any routines to keep your body healthy.

172.   Make sure to save up enough cash so you can retire, as well as some in case you run into health problems. It's important to have money to spare for health problems.

173.   Make sure you prepare for an emergency. As you age you can't move as quickly as you did when you were younger, and it might take you longer to get things together or remember things in a pinch. Have some things in place for when there's an emergency and you need to act fast.

174.   Exercise can improve the aging process. As we get older, our muscle mass naturally declines, making everyday activities more difficult and reducing the number of calories we burn. While aerobic exercise helps maintain muscle mass and

control weight, resistance exercise has the added benefit of helping maintain bone mass.

175. Surround yourself with wonderful people. If you find that the people that you spend a majority of your time with are grouchy more often than they are happy, consider looking for a new group of friends to hang out with. Happiness is contagious and if you are surrounded by it, you are likely to be joyful as well.

176. It is natural to lose some abilities as we age. There is a point in time when someone cannot care for their self. Research local nursing homes, assisted living facilities and retirement communities to find the right place for you. While not the ideal situation for some, in actuality this might be the best available option. There are a variety of different licensed care facilities and professionals who will help assist people who are unable to care for themselves.

177. One of the first things to start going when you age is your eyesight. As you age, it begins to rapidly deteriorate. Make sure that as you age you have frequent visits to the ophthalmologist, in order to track your eyes' degradation, and have

glasses or contacts prescribed in order to make it less drastic.

178.   Do not get stuck in your old ways. The world is changing around you and to think that things will never change is just plain foolish. Evolve to meet the changes and embrace them. Accepting these changes can lead to wonderful adventures for you even through your golden years.

179.   Get fish oils into your life! If not fish oils, then olive, flax or nut oils. These oils have been shown to really improve your health while aging compared to their alternatives like soybean, corn or sunflower oils. The latter oils are processed oils and have been shown to be less healthy for you.

180.   Wonderful memories will be produced by getting out of the house and traveling. You may not have the budget or the health to go on long vacations but just getting out of the house and going to the mall, park or theater is going to make you feel like life is worth living.

181.   Do not let others make you feel as if you are less of a person now than you were in your youth. You may require more care from others

than you used to but you are just as important and it is crucial that you remember who you were and who you are for the rest of your life.

182.   Prepare for the end. If you take the time to prepare a living will and pre-plan your funeral you will find much peace in the process. Dying is a part of living that cannot be beat and having a plan that is ready for that time is a gift to yourself as well as the rest of your family.

183.   Take additional calcium supplements with your vitamins. Calcium gets more important to your body the older that you get. Most adults need about 1,200 mg of calcium each day. If you do not get the amount that your body needs, your bones are going to get brittle and weak.

184.   It is important to take good care of the eyes as you age. Some decrease in your vision is natural with aging, but regular eye exams can detect any serious conditions before they do too much damage.

185.   Keep a positive outlook on life! If you stay positive, your body will be under a lot less stress. The less stress your body is under, the healthier your body will be, the healthier you'll look, and

the longer you'll live. So whenever things get gloomy, try and look at things in a positive light.

186.   We are an optimistic people, always looking to the future. But in old age a backward look, even regret, can be a good thing. Assessing what is good or bad, what worked well or did not, is part of our job as human beings; part of what we pass on to the next generation.

187.   Antioxidants are absolutely one of your best weapons against aging! It is a proven fact that antioxidants counteract the free radicals that are constantly working against your body and the good things you are trying to do with it. Get plenty of antioxidants as you age, with dark vegetables and fruits like carrots, squash and spinach or blue and purple berries!

188.   Have regular eye exams. As you get older, you have to start paying special attention to the health of your eyes, which may be new for you if you have never worn glasses. Reduced eye function can decrease your independence and make it hard to do things you used to do, so have a doctor examine them regularly.

189.   As you age, continue learning. It has never been easier to enroll in a community college or

take classes online. You are never too old to take up a new hobby, study a foreign language, understand statistics, learn about quantum physics or learn anything of interest to you. Lifelong learning will keep your mind sharp and give you goals.

190. The most prevalent cause of hearing loss is aging. Hearing loss is also insidious. It happens so gradually that a person may be hard of hearing without realizing it. If you have not had your hearing tested, you should have a hearing checkup at least by the age of 50.

191. Grab a fashionable pair of sunglasses and wear them. Wearing a cute pair of glasses can help with looking younger but the biggest benefit is the protection it gives to your eyes and skin. The skin around our eyes is very thin and the suns UV rays can do a number on that area. Wearing glasses with that protect from uv rays will keep your skin protected and your eyes bright.

192. Aging shouldn't be a time to sit around and grow old! This is your time to enjoy life and experience new things! Do something you always wanted to do. Take a cruise, go to Vegas, write a

book! Even a new pet can bring new joy and be a positive learning experience!

193.   Taking care of your skin does not only mean using caution when in the sun. You should also take the time to exfoliate your face and body regularly. This gets rid of all of the dry, dead skin that is all over your body which prevents new skin cells from being able to generate in a healthy way.

194.   Get enough sleep. A night's sleep of 7 to 9 hours is crucial to maintaining your hormones, so that you can wake up feeling refreshed. A lack of sleep will more you irritable and stressed making it difficult to enjoy your life to the fullest.

195.   One of the hardest things to manage for the person who is aging and for those around him or her is dementia. If someone you love, has dementia be as patient as possible with them. Often, they don't know the severity of their own condition. To help your own spirits, take their dementia as a mercy, as it must be hard to die having all your memories intact.

196.   You will get a boost from good friends and positive energy. Age is irrelevant when it comes to forming new friendships. Get out there and

meet new people and develop friendships that will help you live a long, wonderful life.

197.   When you get older, it is important to know who you are and what you like. When you focus on what you like, and keep things around you positive, you accent the good things you have going in your life, and will not allow any negative emotions or situations to bring you down.

198.   As you get older, it's more important than ever to surround yourself with people that make you happy, lift you up and do not bring you down. This can be accomplished by having a nice family dinner where everyone is involved or sharing good times and good memories with your favorite people.

199.   Oral health is essential to a long life. Even if you do not have teeth anymore, it is still important to go and have regular exams at the dentist so he can check your gums. You can still develop gum disease, oral cancer and other things that can lead to other health problems.

200.   The appearance of your skin is a key element to looking and feeling younger, so take care of your skin by using moisturizers. This will keep the skin hydrated and soft. Sometimes it will help

to work with a professional dermatologist to determine the right type of lotion and moisturizer that is best for you.

201.   To slow down the aging process, exercise is extremely important. By exercising several times a week, you will help your body keep its muscle strength, stamina, balance and bone density. It is important to include cardio routines as well as strength training sessions, in order to keep the aging process from going too fast.

202.   Stop putting junk into your body as you age for optimum health and greater energy! Although chemicals and preservatives are no good for us at any age, they are a greater burden to an aging body so bring your glasses to the grocery store, read those labels and stop buying things with artificial junk in them that will only work against you!

203.   A tip for staying young, even when your body is aging, is to keep learning. Learn more about playing bridge, how to use a computer, gardening, woodworking, or whatever you wanted to learn earlier in life but didn't have the time to do. Since you are retired and your children are grown, you no longer have the excuse of not having the time to delve into these

new adventures of learning. Never let your brain remain idle!

204.	One of the easiest ways to get more out of life and enjoy life more is to turn off the television. How much time is wasted sitting in front of a television and not living life? It is the same as shorting your life by sitting in front of the idiot box not out enjoying life.

205.	Menopause is a fact of life for aging women. There are many different ways to help relieve the symptoms of menopause and what works for one woman may not work for another. The best thing that you can do is mentally prepare yourself and convince yourself that it is a natural transition that every woman experiences. This will get you in the right frame of mind to deal with menopause.

206.	As your eyes age, you need to take care of them. At the age of 40, have a complete eye exam that will screen for glaucoma, fully measure the vision in each eye, and have your retinas tested for retinal damage. If the findings indicate, be sure to have an annual checkup to make sure that glaucoma or macular eye disease has not begun to show symptoms.

207.   If you are worried about aging then try to do things that will make you feel young again. Go to the mini golf course, or play a few games at the arcade. By doing those things which make you feel young you can actually help slow down the process of aging.

208.   Increasing your social activities can improve your lifestyle as you get older. Being part of a group can help you to keep learning and experiencing new things. Join a seniors group, a craft class, or a cooking class. Keeping busy will give you no time to feel older!

209.   Cultivating solid relationships is essential at all stages of life, but especially when you are aging. Active involvement in the community has been tied to both a longer and a healthier life. Focusing on those who you can emotionally depend on is the best part of social interactions.

210.   In order to age gracefully, be sure to see your doctor regularly! Putting off appointments with your doctor could really be detrimental in your overall health. Regular checkups make is possible for your doctor to catch problems while they are small enough to fix. Save yourself a good bit of time, money and grief by keeping those appointments.

211.   Make sure you are sleeping the number of hours you need. A general rule of thumb for keeping your hormones in check is 7-9 hours per night. Running on too little sleep also makes you grouchy and annoying to be around.

212.   When aging, there is nothing more important than your personal health. If you feel good, consider what you have been doing and find ways to continue the momentum. If you feel mediocre, look for ways you can personally improve your health. If you feel sick, seek help and do so right away.

213.   If you want a tasty way to reduce the risk of osteoporosis, try adding soy to your diet. Soy contains calcium and plant estrogens which help prevent the loss of bone density. You can use soy flour in your favorite recipes, snack on soy nuts, or use soy milk and cheeses.

214.   Oral health is essential to a long life. Even if you do not have teeth anymore, it is still important to go and have regular exams at the dentist so he can check your gums. You can still develop gum disease, oral cancer and other things that can lead to other health problems.

215.   If you're getting up there in age, try asking your doctor about anti-aging supplements. These are special vitamins and minerals that will give your body extra tools to keep you looking and feeling young. But they're not right for everyone, so check with your doctor before you start taking them.

216.   Reflect on life. As you start to get on in years, it is a good idea to reflect on your life and what has worked and not gone so well for you. Take this time to forgive those who have wronged you and to make amends to people you have wronged.

217.   There are 19 foods that are considered to be must have items in your refrigerator and pantry, and they will work wonders for your health and vitality as you age. Write these down and post it somewhere in your home to keep yourself reminded to stay stocked: seafood, dairy, spinach, nuts, olive oil, broccoli, oatmeal, flax seed meal, avocados, pomegranate juice, tomatoes, tofu, yogurt, red onions, garlic, beans and lentils! It may seem like a lot but it is the least you can do for yourself and the best results you can yield from your meal planning efforts!

218. Getting older can often seem like a scary prospect especially for people who are worried about their mental capabilities. The loss of mental ability is a real threat and to help avoid this it is important to maintain a good diet as well as do things to stimulate your thoughts and your brain.

219. As you age, start increasing your intake of raw fruits, seeds, grains, nuts and vegetables. Eat a well balanced diet and be sure to include raw broccoli, cauliflower, soybeans (edamame) and cabbage in your diet. Limit your red meat consumption and try to eat more fish. Raw foods will help your digestion and nutrient absorption.

220. Using olive oil is a key to keep your body looking and feeling young. Olive oil is a versatile, delicious and healthy way to reap the benefits of good oil for your body. Over the years, oils have gotten a bad rap from nutritionists, but oils are essential for keeping a body healthy.

221. A key tip to staying young and healthy is to eat nuts. Nuts are a great snack and a fantastic food to prevent the signs of aging. Nuts are loaded with anti-aging fats and are great sources of dietary fiber, vitamins and minerals. Just be

careful when eating nuts to eat them in moderation because they are high in calories.

222.   Common causes of hearing loss while aging are tinnitus and prebycusis. Tinnitus can be diagnosed by a buzzing or ringing in the ears and prebycusis is just a gradual hearing loss due to aging. Adults over the age of fifty are more prone to prebycusis and tinnitus. Hearing loss is quite common and can be combated by regular ear check-ups and hearing aids.

223.   To minimize the amount of wrinkles that you have, make an effort not to frown. As crazy as it make sound it's really true. Distract yourself when you find yourself frowning by pinching your arm skin instead. Finally, you will be free of the horrible habit.

224.   Switch away from real dairy to dairy substitutes like soy or almond milk. There have been quite a few studies linking dairy products with aging skin. If you want to avoid wrinkles as you age, put down the dairy. The substitutes that are on the market are healthy and tasty so give them a shot.

225.   Did you know that high blood pressure, heart disease and diabetes are risk factors for

dementia? These risks become more severe due to smoking, lack of exercise and high cholesterol. As we age, it becomes increasingly important to control these disorders in order to maintain good mental health as aging progresses.

226.   For healthy aging, don't be afraid to be a bit of a nester. Find things that you absolutely love and put them all around you, whether it's flowers, friends, family, music, movies or any of a multitude of hobbies. When it comes down to it, your home is your place of comfort. Make it your own. Make it a place where you love to be.

227.   Have your hormone levels checked regularly as you age. You will want to have your doctor run standardized tests to be sure that your levels are where they should be. Taking hormone replacement or supplements may be the fix to the way that you have been feeling if you have been feeling bad.

228.   Shake up your life to lead a healthier one. Just because you're aging doesn't mean you can't shake things up, in fact it's healthy to do so. It stimulates your mind and keeps you physically active. This can help improve your mood, your fitness level and your overall health, so don't be

afraid to take a step outside of your normal zone of comfort!

229.   Reduce the amount of stress that you put on yourself. You do not have to do everything for everyone in your life. If the people in your life have learned to depend on you for things that they could very well do on their own, let them do it themselves more often. Then you can relax more.

230.   Stay active during the aging process. Staying active helps your body, mind, and soul. It will help you to age gracefully. Many studies also show that remaining active can have a positive effect on your mental capacity, and may help to keep diseases like Alzheimer's at bay. Try to include activity as part of your daily routine.

231.   Staying properly hydrated has never been more important to you than now! Aging is hard on the body and providing it with plenty of water will help flush toxins, bring nutrients to cells, hydrate skin and make it easier on every function of your body! Most experts recommend about eight glasses of water each day, so drink up for healthier aging!

232.   As you get age, so does your brain. Studies have shown that exercising your brain is as important as exercising your body. Memory exercises will improve the mind and help stave off memory illness or dementia. Small exercises like memorizing 10 objects as you take a walk through your neighborhood, then writing them down when you get home is a good example to the mind nimble and alert.

233.   Make sure you have a good time! Now that you are older, you are free to do exactly what you want, and can make anything happen! Embrace the changes and advantages that come with age and make the most of them.

234.   A tip for staying young, even when your body is aging, is to keep learning. Learn more about playing bridge, how to use a computer, gardening, woodworking, or whatever you wanted to learn earlier in life but didn't have the time to do. Since you are retired and your children are grown, you no longer have the excuse of not having the time to delve into these new adventures of learning. Never let your brain remain idle!

235.   Make your home easier to get around in. Remove rugs and other things you can easily slip

on. Place things where you can reach them. Get clocks with larger numbers. By making your home easier to live in, you can relax instead of struggling to do things you once did. Adapt, and growing older will be easier.

236.   A key tip to staying young and healthy is to eat nuts. Nuts are a great snack and a fantastic food to prevent the signs of aging. Nuts are loaded with anti-aging fats and are great sources of dietary fiber, vitamins and minerals. Just be careful when eating nuts to eat them in moderation because they are high in calories.

237.   If you are retired, try to find outlets to keep you involved in your community and keep friendships. Local schools often need volunteers, contact local schools in your area if this sounds like something fun for you to do. Keeping a social life can help fight off depression which sometimes can become overwhelming if you are on your own.

238.   Common causes of hearing loss while aging are tinnitus and prebycusis. Tinnitus can be diagnosed by a buzzing or ringing in the ears and prebycusis is just a gradual hearing loss due to aging. Adults over the age of fifty are more prone to prebycusis and tinnitus. Hearing loss is

quite common and can be combated by regular ear check-ups and hearing aids.

239.   Moisturizing regularly will help reduce unwanted wrinkling and other signs of aging that become visible on our skin. You want to choose a moisturizing routine that will keep your skin hydrated. Check with a dermatologist to see what will work for you the best and make sure to use it on a regular basis. They don't do much good in the bottle.

240.   Learn a new language, play Sudoku, travel the world! These are all things that can help you stay younger longer. Challenging yourself mentally has been shown to keep your brain younger. Audit some classes at the local college or just start up a book club with your friends. Keep your brain active and engaged!

241.   If your health is good, be sure to preserve it. If it is not so good, do what you can to improve it. Your body is your life vessel and should be cared for as if your life depends on it, because it does. Get the help that you need to improve any health issues that you may have.

242.   In order to keep your body from aging it is very important that you get the right amount of

sleep. For most people, the way they look is largely dependent on how much sleep they get. Having eight hours of sleep every night is ideal but it varies from person to person.

243.   Prepare for the end. If you take the time to prepare a living will and pre-plan your funeral you will find much peace in the process. Dying is a part of living that cannot be beat and having a plan that is ready for that time is a gift to yourself as well as the rest of your family.

244.   While an occasional drink every now and then is perfectly acceptable, in order to slow the aging process, alcohol is something that should be avoided. In excess, alcohol can cause cardiovascular diseases, certain cancers, can weaken your immune system and affect your system of balance resulting in injuries. By limiting alcohol, you are helping your body fight the inevitable aging process.

245.   Pay special attention to your diet. As you get older, you need to pay attention to what you are eating much more carefully. A balanced diet is essential to keep as healthy and energized as possible. Try to eat 5 servings of fruits and vegetables, and 3 servings of whole grains per day. Limit your fat intake to no more than 30

percent of your diet. Focus on complex carbohydrates, such as wild rice, whole wheat bread and oatmeal. Last but not least, drink plenty of water.

246.   Try moving around more and sitting still less. Especially if you're retired and aren't moving around for work any more. Try taking up a hobby that involves moving around - golf is a particularly good once since it's not a high impact sport but it keeps you moving. Studies have shown that getting up and moving can help you keep your blood pressure levels in normal ranges and lower your risk for heart problems.

247.   A key tip to staying young and healthy is to eat nuts. Nuts are a great snack and a fantastic food to prevent the signs of aging. Nuts are loaded with anti-aging fats and are great sources of dietary fiber, vitamins and minerals. Just be careful when eating nuts to eat them in moderation because they are high in calories.

248.   To combat the aging process one of the things that you can do is get some sun. This will help you to maximize the way that you feel and get vitamin D into your system, which can be very beneficial for your looks. During the spring

and summer, spend at least an hour in the sun to look much younger and feel great during the day.

249.   Consider volunteering with a church or community organization to keep yourself active and to expand your circle of friends and acquaintances. Many organizations rely heavily on volunteers and you can frequently find one supporting a cause or work you believe in. As an additional benefit, volunteering exposes you to others with similar interests, making it easier to find new friends or peers.

250.   During the course of the day, act silly and joke around with friends and family. The more that you joke, the lower your heart rate will be and the better you will feel as the day wears on. This can go a long way in reducing your stress and helping you to become more beautiful.

251.   Most people lose some degree of their hearing as they grow older. This may not present a problem for you yet. However, it is important to know how sharp your hearing is because it greatly affects your quality of life. If you find yourself missing what others say, asking them to repeat themselves, or turning up the radio or TV, you may be at risk for hearing loss and should have it checked immediately.

252.   When you wake up in the morning, find the newspaper and pull out the daily crossword puzzle. Keeping your mind active and sharp can improve your brain activity, which will combat the signs of aging mentally. Also, you will be able to stay alert and participate in conversations with friends and family.

253.   Many people gain weight as they age. You can decrease the chances of diabetes, high blood pressure, and select cancers by having a healthy weight. Eating healthy food and exercising will help your body maintain a healthy weight.

254.   Determine how much sleep your body needs a night and then make sure you get it. Lack of good regular sleep is a possible cause of premature aging. Just because you're getting older does not mean that you need less sleep. Our bodies function better when they have had a full nights sleep. Studies have shown that it is very hard to recover from a sleep deficit so keep to a pattern as much as possible.

255.   Do not leave the house without sunscreen to avoid looking older faster. The UV radiation from the sun can severely damage your skin and it is a major contributor to how your face looks.

Also know that too much sun exposure can lead to certain cancers so wear sunscreen every day.

256.   One of the hardest things to manage for the person who is aging and for those around him or her is dementia. If someone you love, has dementia be as patient as possible with them. Often, they don't know the severity of their own condition. To help your own spirits, take their dementia as a mercy, as it must be hard to die having all your memories intact.

257.   You will get a boost from good friends and positive energy. No one is ever too old to begin new friendships. Go and find new friends. It can help you live longer and have a more fulfilled life.

258.   When you get older, it is important to know who you are and what you like. When you focus on what you like, and keep things around you positive, you accent the good things you have going in your life, and will not allow any negative emotions or situations to bring you down.

259.   You know you should eat healthy as you age to keep your body in optimum health. Every once in a while, though, you need to indulge yourself. This way, you do not have to dread the

same old same old every day, and can look forward to this treat. This may help you keep to your healthier eating plan if you know you get to have a party occasionally.

260.   Do not let others make you feel as if you are less of a person now than you were in your youth. You may require more care from others than you used to but you are just as important and it is crucial that you remember who you were and who you are for the rest of your life.

261.   Avoid exposing your skin to extreme weather conditions. The cold air and the sun can both equally damage your skin. It can increase your risk of premature aging of the skin as well as more serious problems, including skin cancer.

262.   Keep a positive outlook on life! If you stay positive, your body will be under a lot less stress. The less stress your body is under, the healthier your body will be, the healthier you'll look, and the longer you'll live. So whenever things get gloomy, try and look at things in a positive light.

263.   Smoothies are a great and delicious way to get more nutrients as we age! You can combine literally anything to create a tasty treat that delivers valuable vitamins and minerals to your

system. Add fruits, vegetables, flax seeds and yogurt or ice-cream to mix a potent potion you can enjoy any time of the day!

264.   Maintain a positive attitude. You're only as old as you feel, and if you stay positive aging can be a wonderful time of your life. Make sure you start every day giving thanks for what you have in your life, and watch how much better the day is when you approach it happily.

265.   Go out with friends and family. One of the worst things to do as you start to get older is to isolate yourself in your home. Make sure you get out a few times a week for anything: to volunteer, to have lunch or any of hundreds of possibilities. Going out and seeing others has a great effect on your mental health.

266.   As you become older you will start to find parts of your body not working as well as they used to. For some things, it is possible to take medication but for others, you will simply have to accept these facts. It can be hard to accept but the faster you do the easier it will be for you.

267.   In order to look and feel young, doing some strength training every other day is a key. People who have toned, strong muscles always look

younger than their years. Not much is necessary in order to see the benefits of strength training, just twenty minutes every other day can lead to a toned and more youthful appearance.

268.   The key to enjoy aging is to accept it. Instead of focusing on creaky bones and reduced vision, give attention to the joy of growing more in love with your partner and playing with your grandchildren. Like everything else in life, learn to focus on the positives to enjoy life more.

269.   As you age, continue learning. It has never been easier to enroll in a community college or take classes online. You are never too old to take up a new hobby, study a foreign language, understand statistics, learn about quantum physics or learn anything of interest to you. Lifelong learning will keep your mind sharp and give you goals.

270.   Drink water! Water is one of the most vital things for you to drink - as the day wears on - if you want to combat aging. Try to drink at least eight glasses of water a day, spread it out , drink in the morning, afternoon and evening. This will make you feel better and improve the quality of your skin tone too!

271.   Sugar has been proven to have an aging affect. You don't have to cut it out of your life completely, but definitely cut back on it. It has been shown to actually reduce the lifespan in multiple studies. Stick with foods that are naturally sweet like fruits to help your sweet cravings.

272.   Work with some weights to keep yourself looking younger. A toned body is a young body no matter what the chronological age may say. Working with the appropriate weights for your health will help you keep your body toned and looking fit, which will take years off of your body and soul.

273.   Go nuts with nuts! Nuts are one of the worlds most perfect foods. They are filled with important vitamins, minerals and fats that help our bodies stay in the best shape they can be. They are a great snack food as they really help us fill up without having to eat a lot of them. Be careful with them though as they are high in calories.

274.   Let guilt go. A long life is sure to have things that you may feel guilty about. Do not let this guilt run your life. Make amends or forgive yourself and forget. In many cases there is no

way to undo the things that have been done, and all that we can do is make the most of the time we have left.

275.   Focus on the quality of your life and stop worrying about statistics. Your doctors are paid for worrying about height, age, and weight. Dwelling on age, weight and looks can make you miss out on important events and opportunities.

276.   In order to age gracefully, be sure to see your doctor regularly! Putting off appointments with your doctor could really be detrimental in your overall health. Regular checkups make is possible for your doctor to catch problems while they are small enough to fix. Save yourself a good bit of time, money and grief by keeping those appointments.

277.   Get a tea break into your daily routine. Teas have some fabulous benefits when it comes to age prevention. They are chock full of healthy antioxidants and other cancer-battling ingredients. Plus the break itself can be an amazing stress reliever in its own right. Tea breaks are one of the healthiest habits you can form!

278.   Do some housecleaning with your social contacts. It has been proven that smiling and laughing have the ability to decrease wrinkle formation, allowing you to look young longer. Spend as much time as possible doing things you enjoy with people who make you laugh.

279.   Exercise is necessary for healthy aging. Regular exercise can delay or prevent heart disease and Diabetes as well as lessen the pain of Arthritis, depression and anxiety. Four kinds should be followed: aerobics to build endurance and keep your heart and blood vessels healthy; strength training to reduce age-related loss of muscle; stretching to keep your body flexible; and balance exercises to reduce your chances of falling.

280.   The appearance of your skin is a key element to looking and feeling younger, so take care of your skin by using moisturizers. This will keep the skin hydrated and soft. Sometimes it will help to work with a professional dermatologist to determine the right type of lotion and moisturizer that is best for you.

281.   As you get age, so does your brain. Studies have shown that exercising your brain is as important as exercising your body. Memory

exercises will improve the mind and help stave off memory illness or dementia. Small exercises like memorizing 10 objects as you take a walk through your neighborhood, then writing them down when you get home is a good example to the mind nimble and alert.

282.   Maintain a positive attitude. You're only as old as you feel, and if you stay positive aging can be a wonderful time of your life. Make sure you start every day giving thanks for what you have in your life, and watch how much better the day is when you approach it happily.

283.   As people age, muscle tone is compromised naturally. If you have jiggly skin between your elbows to armpits you will want to try to tone that area before it is too late to do anything about it. Getting rid of this type of flab can be done using very light weights and modified push ups.

284.   One simple tip to take care of your eyes as they age is to apply a compress for five minutes, made of a washcloth wrung out in hot water. The compress will clear your eyes of "sleep" and other bacterial material that can contribute to eye infections and diseases as you age.

285. Most people lose some degree of their hearing as they grow older. This may not present a problem for you yet. However, it is important to know how sharp your hearing is because it greatly affects your quality of life. If you find yourself missing what others say, asking them to repeat themselves, or turning up the radio or TV, you may be at risk for hearing loss and should have it checked immediately.

286. Thinning hair is quite common with aging. It can happen due to medications, hereditary conditions, menopause or illness. Thinning hair can be an irritating thing to deal with and you may talk to your doctor about your options. There are many hair extensions on the market today which will hide the problem without the use of old fashioned wigs.

287. Exercise can improve the aging process. As we get older, our muscle mass naturally declines, making everyday activities more difficult and reducing the number of calories we burn. While aerobic exercise helps maintain muscle mass and control weight, resistance exercise has the added benefit of helping maintain bone mass.

288. Developing good coping skills can improve the aging process. Finding the silver lining

around the clouds in your life has been associated with a longer life. If you are not naturally an optimist, it's never too late to change. By focusing on the positive in your life, you can be positive you will age better.

289.   When you get older, it is important to know who you are and what you like. When you focus on what you like, and keep things around you positive, you accent the good things you have going in your life, and will not allow any negative emotions or situations to bring you down.

290.   When the years are beginning to creep up on you, look at them with joy and not sadness, and spread your wisdom to those around you. You will get a good sense of satisfaction knowing that you have spread this joy to others. It is a great gift, and one that does not have to cost a penny.

291.   If you find that you are feeling lonely when you are at home, consider getting a pet. They are wonderful companions and will provide you with company when no one else is around. Be sure that you pick the pet that will work out the best for you. If you do not want to commit to just one pet, consider being a foster home for animals in shelters.

292.   Stop multitasking! Your mind cannot function the way that it once did. You will find it easier and far less stressful if you do not try to accomplish as many things at once. Avoiding stress is important as you get older to avoid doing damage to your heart and your body.

293.   Make sure you're only drinking alcohol in moderation. For those under 65, this means you shouldn't drink more than two glasses a day. If you're over 65, this means you shouldn't drink more than one glass a day. If you're going to drink alcohol try drinking wine instead since it's shown to benefit health in small doses, unlike beer or hard liqueur.

294.   Eating small amounts of food more often during the day instead of big, heavy meals all at once, will work wonders for your entire system, and help you to control weight gain as you age! Your ability to absorb nutrients is greatly aided by frequent, small portions of food and can also cut down on your heartburn. So plan these mini-meals out in advance and stick to the program. Your body will thank you for it!

295.   You will have less of a chance to get a heart disease if you eat less red meat and more fish. There are many unhealthy fats in red meat that

can contribute to clogging of the arteries, and this can result in heart disease, as well as other illnesses. While fish, on the other hand, does the opposite. Adding it to your meals and reducing the amount of red meat that you eat will help you to have a healthier and longer life.

296.   Although everyone misplaces things and forgets things from time to time, no matter how old you are, if you notice that you or a loved on started being overly forgetful or misplaces items in strange places, it is time to talk to a doctor. Frequently forgetting things or placing everyday objects such as your car keys in the microwave or freezer is a cause for concern.

297.   As you age, continue learning. It has never been easier to enroll in a community college or take classes online. You are never too old to take up a new hobby, study a foreign language, understand statistics, learn about quantum physics or learn anything of interest to you. Lifelong learning will keep your mind sharp and give you goals.

298.   It is important to have your blood pressure read on a regular basis. If you have high blood pressure you may not even know it, that is why they call it the 'silent killer'. You will have to be

careful to have your blood pressure checked often since your cardiovascular system works less effectively as you grow older. If you discover any problems, you can deal with them immediately.

299.   When your body ages, the need for down time increases, which means you must get adequate sleep. Try to have a set time for going to bed, which allows you to get comfortable and fall asleep at a reasonable time. Read a book or magazine to help induce sleepiness, however, the TV should be avoided because of the stimulation it can cause.

300.   So, you have been looking in the mirror? Wanting to look younger and feel good? This will give you motivation you need. Improve your body mass index by shedding off a few unwanted pounds in the upcoming month. Keep a positive mindset, and improve your outlook on life at the same time!

301.   Think about doing volunteer work after you retire. This will make your days more fulfilling and interesting. In addition, it will extend your social network. Non-profits are always looking for volunteers, and they often do not get enough. If you can volunteer your time, you will be providing them with a very valuable service.

302.   Keeping your weight under control is one key to aging well. There are a number of ailments related to obesity which exacerbate age-related illnesses. In order to keep your weight under control, you should exercise moderately and eat a balanced diet. Tracking your food intake with an online food diary makes this easier.

303.   Keeping your cholesterol under control is important for aging well. A build up of cholesterol can raise your risk of stroke or heart attack. Eating a diet low in animal fats and high in fiber can help keep your cholesterol level under control by increasing your HDL (good) cholesterol and reducing your LDL (bad) cholesterol.

304.   Try eating more resveratrol. Resveratrol mimics the natural processes related to calorie restriction diets. Resveratrol can be found in nuts and grapes and can also have an anti aging effect. Resvestrol can be found in knotweed, a Japanese root that is the main source of resveratrol companies use for supplements. It is also present in high levels in Senna quinquangulata, which is a common shrub native to South America.

305.   For healthy aging, consider grazing over six smaller meals, instead of three big ones. Studies have shown that this helps your body absorb more nutrients, control its weight and decrease the potential for heartburn. In fact, some studies have shown that eating the same amount of calories in six smaller meals has led to considerable weight loss!

306.   Feel free to have a drink and a good meal once in a while. Even if you are watching your diet closely and do not consume alcohol on a regular basis, you should take the time to have a good glass of wine that you used to love and a great meal that was your favorite. Enjoy things in life.

307.   Eat more nuts throughout the day. Nuts are a great food to help prevent aging. They have many healthy vitamins, minerals and fats, which will help balance your daily nutrition. Plus, they are an excellent way to stop your processed food cravings between meals, leading you to a much healthier lifestyle!

308.   Progress feels good for everyone. If you find things to accomplish every day, you are going to feel great when you accomplish them. Find problems to solve. This could be helping

someone who needs the help or just completing a simple jigsaw puzzle. The accomplishment will feel great, either way.

309.   While it is probably something one would rather not think about as one ages, it can be beneficial to be aware of one's mortality. In what sense? The purpose of this is not to dwell on the "end", but rather to make us realize that every day is important, and that life is a gift we should take advantage of in every capacity.

310.   Take additional calcium supplements with your vitamins. Calcium gets more important to your body the older that you get. Most adults need about 1,200 mg of calcium each day. If you do not get the amount that your body needs, your bones are going to get brittle and weak.

311.   Make sure you're keeping active. Your body needs exercise to function properly, especially as you age. Adding thirty minutes of exercise into your daily routine can not only keep you looking younger, but it can also extend your life. And don't wait until you're already old to exercise, start as early as possible.

312.   Make sure you're getting enough vitamin D in your diet. If you're not, try eating more fish or

drinking more milk. If you can't do either of those, look into supplements. Vitamin D has been shown to slow the aging process and can keep you looking and feeling young much longer. Plus, it has other health benefits as well!

313.   Get quality sleep on a regular basis to keep your body balanced and better equipped to age gracefully! Many people of all ages suffer from lack of sleep and poor quality of it and it is even more important to us as we get older. Seek medical advice if you are not getting the sleep you need and do not underestimate the importance of it to you!

314.   Maintain a positive attitude. You're only as old as you feel, and if you stay positive aging can be a wonderful time of your life. Make sure you start every day giving thanks for what you have in your life, and watch how much better the day is when you approach it happily.

315.   Write your life story down. It doesn't have to be a major novel, but create some account of your life so that your children or grandchildren can get to know all of the things you've seen and gone through during your life. No children? Do it for relatives or friends.

316.   As people age, muscle tone is compromised naturally. If you have jiggly skin between your elbows to armpits you will want to try to tone that area before it is too late to do anything about it. Getting rid of this type of flab can be done using very light weights and modified push ups.

317.   The skin naturally looses its elasticity as people age. Sometimes aging people notice baggy knees as a part of this process. Baggy knees can be combated with simple shallow squats to help strengthen the quadriceps. Do not overdo it and begin slowly with two sets. As you become more skilled, add another set. Do the squats daily.